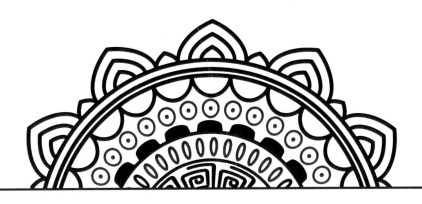

THIS JOURNAL BELONGS TO :

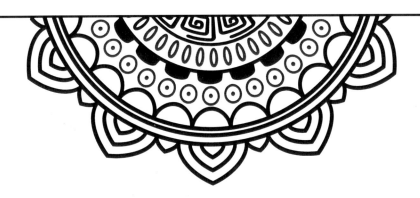

YOGA LESSON PLAN

Venue :		Date / Time :	
Lesson Plan Ref :			
Level :		Lesson Duration :	

Lesson Objectives :

Sequence :

Props / Oils :	Music :

Quote:

*" Yoga is not about self-improvement.
It's about self-acceptance."*

YOGA LESSON PLAN

Venue :		Date / Time :	
Lesson Plan Ref :			
Level :		Lesson Duration :	

Lesson Objectives :

Sequence :

Props / Oils :	Music :

Quote:

" *Yoga teaches us to cure what need not be endured and endure what cannot be cured* "

YOGA LESSON PLAN

Venue :		Date / Time :	
Lesson Plan Ref :			
Level :		Lesson Duration :	

Lesson Objectives :

Sequence :

Props / Oils :	Music :

Quote:

" Sky above earth below peace within "

YOGA LESSON PLAN

Venue :		Date / Time :	
Lesson Plan Ref :			
Level :		Lesson Duration :	

Lesson Objectives :

Sequence :

Props / Oils :

Music :

Quote:

" The body benefits from movement, and the mind benefits from stillness "

YOGA LESSON PLAN

Venue :		Date / Time :	
Lesson Plan Ref :			
Level :		Lesson Duration :	

Lesson Objectives :

Sequence :

Props / Oils :	Music :

Quote:

" My biggest struggles have been my biggest teachers "

YOGA LESSON PLAN

Venue :		Date / Time :	
Lesson Plan Ref :			
Level :		Lesson Duration :	

Lesson Objectives :

Sequence :

| Props / Oils : | Music : |

Quote:

*" Calming the mind is yoga.
Not just standing on the head "*

YOGA LESSON PLAN

Venue :		Date / Time :	
Lesson Plan Ref :			
Level :		Lesson Duration :	

Lesson Objectives :

Sequence :

Props / Oils :	Music :

Quote:

"The body is your temple. Keep it pure and clean for the soul to reside in"

YOGA LESSON PLAN

Venue :		Date / Time :	
Lesson Plan Ref :			
Level :		Lesson Duration :	

Lesson Objectives :

Sequence :

Props / Oils :

Music :

Quote:

*" Sometimes giving yourself a break
is th very thing you need "*

YOGA LESSON PLAN

Venue :		Date / Time :	
Lesson Plan Ref :			
Level :		Lesson Duration :	

Lesson Objectives :

Sequence :

Props / Oils :

Music :

Quote:

" Yoga does not transform the way we see things, it transforms the person who sees "

YOGA LESSON PLAN

Venue :		Date / Time :	
Lesson Plan Ref :			
Level :		Lesson Duration :	

Lesson Objectives :

Sequence :

Props / Oils :

Music :

Quote:

" Yoga is the perfect opportunity to be curious about who you are"

YOGA LESSON PLAN

Venue :		Date / Time :	
Lesson Plan Ref :			
Level :		Lesson Duration :	

Lesson Objectives :

Sequence :

Props / Oils :

Music :

Quote:

" I bend so I don't break "

YOGA LESSON PLAN

Venue :		Date / Time :	
Lesson Plan Ref :			
Level :		Lesson Duration :	

Lesson Objectives :

Sequence :

Props / Oils :

Music :

Quote:

" Throw your hair in a bun, downward dog like a boss, and handle it "

YOGA LESSON PLAN

Venue :		Date / Time :	
Lesson Plan Ref :			
Level :		Lesson Duration :	

Lesson Objectives :

Sequence :

Props / Oils :	Music :

Quote:

" Inhale the future, exhale the past"

YOGA LESSON PLAN

Venue :		Date / Time :	
Lesson Plan Ref :			
Level :		Lesson Duration :	

Lesson Objectives :

Sequence :

Props / Oils :

Music :

Quote:

" *The pose begins when you want to leave it* "

YOGA LESSON PLAN

Venue :		Date / Time :	
Lesson Plan Ref :			
Level :		Lesson Duration :	

Lesson Objectives :

Sequence :

Props / Oils :

Music :

Quote:

" The longest journey of any person is the journey inward "

YOGA LESSON PLAN

Venue :		Date / Time :	
Lesson Plan Ref :			
Level :		Lesson Duration :	

Lesson Objectives :

Sequence :

Props / Oils :

Music :

Quote:

" Yoga is a mirror to look at ourselves from within "

YOGA LESSON PLAN

Venue :		Date / Time :	
Lesson Plan Ref :			
Level :		Lesson Duration :	

Lesson Objectives :

Sequence :

Props / Oils :

Music :

Quote:

" The yoga pose you avoid the most you need the most"

YOGA LESSON PLAN

Venue :		Date / Time :	
Lesson Plan Ref :			
Level :		Lesson Duration :	

Lesson Objectives :

Sequence :

Props / Oils :

Music :

Quote:

" Yoga is the journey of the self, through the self, to the self "

YOGA LESSON PLAN

Venue :		Date / Time :	
Lesson Plan Ref :			
Level :		Lesson Duration :	

Lesson Objectives :

Sequence :

Props / Oils :	Music :

Quote:

" Yoga is the fountain of youth. You've only as young as your spine is flexible "

YOGA LESSON PLAN

Venue :		Date / Time :	
Lesson Plan Ref :			
Level :		Lesson Duration :	

Lesson Objectives :

Sequence :

Props / Oils :	Music :

Quote:

" A flower does not think of competing to the flower next to it. It just blooms "

YOGA LESSON PLAN

Venue :		Date / Time :	
Lesson Plan Ref :			
Level :		Lesson Duration :	

Lesson Objectives :

Sequence :

Props / Oils :	Music :

Quote:

" *Yoga exists in the world because everything is linked* "

YOGA LESSON PLAN

Venue :		Date / Time :	
Lesson Plan Ref :			
Level :		Lesson Duration :	

Lesson Objectives :

Sequence :

Props / Oils :	Music :

Quote:

" Yoga. Because punching people is frowned upon."

YOGA LESSON PLAN

Venue :		Date / Time :	
Lesson Plan Ref :			
Level :		Lesson Duration :	

Lesson Objectives :

Sequence :

Props / Oils :	Music :

Quote:

" Yoga is not for the flexible. It's for th willing"

YOGA LESSON PLAN

Venue :		Date / Time :	
Lesson Plan Ref :			
Level :		Lesson Duration :	

Lesson Objectives :

Sequence :

Props / Oils :	Music :

Quote:

" For those wounded by civilization, yoga is the most healing salve "

YOGA LESSON PLAN

Venue :		Date / Time :	
Lesson Plan Ref :			
Level :		Lesson Duration :	

Lesson Objectives :

Sequence :

Props / Oils :

Music :

Quote:

" Yoga is the space where flower blossoms."

YOGA LESSON PLAN

Venue :		Date / Time :	
Lesson Plan Ref :			
Level :		Lesson Duration :	

Lesson Objectives :

Sequence :

Props / Oils :	Music :

Quote:

"Yoga is the cessation of the movements of the mind.
Then there is abiding in the Seer's own form."

YOGA LESSON PLAN

Venue :		Date / Time :	
Lesson Plan Ref :			
Level :		Lesson Duration :	

Lesson Objectives :

Sequence :

Props / Oils :	Music :

Quote:

" The attitude of gratitude is the highest yoga. "

YOGA LESSON PLAN

Venue :		Date / Time :	
Lesson Plan Ref :			
Level :		Lesson Duration :	

Lesson Objectives :

Sequence :

Props / Oils :	Music :

Quote:

" The soul is here for its own joy. "

YOGA LESSON PLAN

Venue :		Date / Time :	
Lesson Plan Ref :			
Level :		Lesson Duration :	

Lesson Objectives :

Sequence :

Props / Oils :

Music :

Quote:

" Yoga is 99% practice and 1% theory. "

YOGA LESSON PLAN

Venue :		Date / Time :	
Lesson Plan Ref :			
Level :		Lesson Duration :	

Lesson Objectives :

Sequence :

Props / Oils :

Music :

Quote:

" Here and now is where yoga begins "

YOGA LESSON PLAN

Venue :		Date / Time :	
Lesson Plan Ref :			
Level :		Lesson Duration :	

Lesson Objectives :

Sequence :

Props / Oils :	Music :

Quote:

" Yoga is not about self-improvement.
It's about self-acceptance."

YOGA LESSON PLAN

Venue :		Date / Time :	
Lesson Plan Ref :			
Level :		Lesson Duration :	

Lesson Objectives :

Sequence :

Props / Oils :

Music :

Quote:

" Yoga teaches us to cure what need not be endured and endure what cannot be cured "

YOGA LESSON PLAN

Venue :		Date / Time :	
Lesson Plan Ref :			
Level :		Lesson Duration :	

Lesson Objectives :

Sequence :

Props / Oils :	Music :

Quote:

" Sky above earth below peace within "

YOGA LESSON PLAN

Venue :		Date / Time :	
Lesson Plan Ref :			
Level :		Lesson Duration :	

Lesson Objectives :

Sequence :

Props / Oils :

Music :

Quote:

" The body benefits from movement, and the mind benefits from stillness "

YOGA LESSON PLAN

Venue :		Date / Time :	
Lesson Plan Ref :			
Level :		Lesson Duration :	

Lesson Objectives :

Sequence :

Props / Oils :	Music :

Quote:

" My biggest struggles have been my biggest teachers "

YOGA LESSON PLAN

Venue :		Date / Time :	
Lesson Plan Ref :			
Level :		Lesson Duration :	

Lesson Objectives :

Sequence :

Props / Oils :

Music :

Quote:

*" Calming the mind is yoga.
Not just standing on the head "*

YOGA LESSON PLAN

Venue :		Date / Time :	
Lesson Plan Ref :			
Level :		Lesson Duration :	

Lesson Objectives :

Sequence :

Props / Oils :

Music :

Quote:

"The body is your temple. Keep it pure and clean for the soul to reside in"

YOGA LESSON PLAN

Venue :		Date / Time :	
Lesson Plan Ref :			
Level :		Lesson Duration :	

Lesson Objectives :

Sequence :

Props / Oils :

Music :

Quote:

*" Sometimes giving yourself a break
is th very thing you need "*

YOGA LESSON PLAN

Venue :		Date / Time :	
Lesson Plan Ref :			
Level :		Lesson Duration :	

Lesson Objectives :

Sequence :

Props / Oils :	Music :

Quote:

" Yoga does not transform the way we see things, it transforms the person who sees "

YOGA LESSON PLAN

Venue :		Date / Time :	
Lesson Plan Ref :			
Level :		Lesson Duration :	

Lesson Objectives :

Sequence :

Props / Oils :

Music :

Quote:

" *Yoga is the perfect opportunity to be curious about who you are* "

YOGA LESSON PLAN

Venue :		Date / Time :	
Lesson Plan Ref :			
Level :		Lesson Duration :	

Lesson Objectives :

Sequence :

Props / Oils :

Music :

Quote:

" I bend so I don't break "

YOGA LESSON PLAN

Venue :		Date / Time :	
Lesson Plan Ref :			
Level :		Lesson Duration :	

Lesson Objectives :

Sequence :

Props / Oils :	Music :

Quote:

" Throw your hair in a bun, downward dog like a boss, and handle it "

YOGA LESSON PLAN

Venue :		Date / Time :	
Lesson Plan Ref :			
Level :		Lesson Duration :	

Lesson Objectives :

Sequence :

Props / Oils :	Music :

Quote:

" Inhale the future, exhale the past "

YOGA LESSON PLAN

Venue :		Date / Time :	
Lesson Plan Ref :			
Level :		Lesson Duration :	

Lesson Objectives :

Sequence :

Props / Oils :

Music :

Quote:

" The pose begins when you want to leave it "

YOGA LESSON PLAN

Venue :		Date / Time :	
Lesson Plan Ref :			
Level :		Lesson Duration :	

Lesson Objectives :

Sequence :

Props / Oils :

Music :

Quote:

" The longest journey of any person is the journey inward "

YOGA LESSON PLAN

Venue :		Date / Time :	
Lesson Plan Ref :			
Level :		Lesson Duration :	

Lesson Objectives :

Sequence :

Props / Oils :	Music :

Quote:

" Yoga is a mirror to look at ourselves from within "

YOGA LESSON PLAN

Venue :		Date / Time :	
Lesson Plan Ref :			
Level :		Lesson Duration :	

Lesson Objectives :

Sequence :

Props / Oils :

Music :

Quote:

" The yoga pose you avoid the most you need the most "

YOGA LESSON PLAN

Venue :		Date / Time :	
Lesson Plan Ref :			
Level :		Lesson Duration :	

Lesson Objectives :

Sequence :

Props / Oils :	Music :

Quote:

" Yoga is the journey of the self, through the self, to the self "

YOGA LESSON PLAN

Venue :		Date / Time :	
Lesson Plan Ref :			
Level :		Lesson Duration :	

Lesson Objectives :

Sequence :

Props / Oils :	Music :

Quote:

" Yoga is the fountain of youth. You've only as young as your spine is flexible "

YOGA LESSON PLAN

Venue :		Date / Time :	
Lesson Plan Ref :			
Level :		Lesson Duration :	

Lesson Objectives :

Sequence :

Props / Oils :

Music :

Quote:

" A flower does not think of competing to the flower next to it. It just blooms "

YOGA LESSON PLAN

Venue :		Date / Time :	
Lesson Plan Ref :			
Level :		Lesson Duration :	

Lesson Objectives :

Sequence :

Props / Oils :	Music :

Quote:

" *Yoga exists in the world because everything is linked* "

YOGA LESSON PLAN

Venue :		Date / Time :	
Lesson Plan Ref :			
Level :		Lesson Duration :	

Lesson Objectives :

Sequence :

Props / Oils :

Music :

Quote:

" Yoga. Because punching people is frowned upon."

YOGA LESSON PLAN

Venue :		Date / Time :	
Lesson Plan Ref :			
Level :		Lesson Duration :	

Lesson Objectives :

Sequence :

Props / Oils :

Music :

Quote:

" Yoga is not for the flexible. It's for th willing "

YOGA LESSON PLAN

Venue :		Date / Time :	
Lesson Plan Ref :			
Level :		Lesson Duration :	

Lesson Objectives :

Sequence :

Props / Oils :	Music :

Quote:

" For those wounded by civilization, yoga is the most healing salve "

YOGA LESSON PLAN

Venue :		Date / Time :	
Lesson Plan Ref :			
Level :		Lesson Duration :	

Lesson Objectives :

Sequence :

Props / Oils :	Music :

Quote:

" Yoga is the space where flower blossoms."

YOGA LESSON PLAN

Venue :		Date / Time :	
Lesson Plan Ref :			
Level :		Lesson Duration :	

Lesson Objectives :

Sequence :

Props / Oils :

Music :

Quote:
" Yoga is the cessation of the movements of the mind.
Then there is abiding in the Seer's own form."

YOGA LESSON PLAN

Venue :		Date / Time :	
Lesson Plan Ref :			
Level :		Lesson Duration :	

Lesson Objectives :

Sequence :

Props / Oils :	Music :

Quote:

" The attitude of gratitude is the highest yoga. "

YOGA LESSON PLAN

Venue :		Date / Time :	
Lesson Plan Ref :			
Level :		Lesson Duration :	

Lesson Objectives :

Sequence :

Props / Oils :

Music :

Quote:

" The soul is here for its own joy. "

YOGA LESSON PLAN

Venue :		Date / Time :	
Lesson Plan Ref :			
Level :		Lesson Duration :	

Lesson Objectives :

Sequence :

Props / Oils :	Music :

Quote:

" Yoga is 99% practice and 1% theory. "

YOGA LESSON PLAN

Venue :		Date / Time :	
Lesson Plan Ref :			
Level :		Lesson Duration :	

Lesson Objectives :

Sequence :

Props / Oils :	Music :

Quote:

" Here and now is where yoga begins "

YOGA LESSON PLAN

Venue :		Date / Time :	
Lesson Plan Ref :			
Level :		Lesson Duration :	

Lesson Objectives :

Sequence :

Props / Oils :	Music :

Quote:

" Yoga is not about self-improvement.
It's about self-acceptance."

YOGA LESSON PLAN

Venue :		Date / Time :	
Lesson Plan Ref :			
Level :		Lesson Duration :	

Lesson Objectives :

Sequence :

Props / Oils :	Music :

Quote:

" Yoga teaches us to cure what need not be endured and endure what cannot be cured "

YOGA LESSON PLAN

Venue :		Date / Time :	
Lesson Plan Ref :			
Level :		Lesson Duration :	

Lesson Objectives :

Sequence :

Props / Oils :	Music :

Quote:

" Sky above earth below peace within "

YOGA LESSON PLAN

Venue :		Date / Time :	
Lesson Plan Ref :			
Level :		Lesson Duration :	

Lesson Objectives :

Sequence :

Props / Oils :

Music :

Quote:

*" The body benefits from movement,
and the mind benefits from stillness "*

YOGA LESSON PLAN

Venue :		Date / Time :	
Lesson Plan Ref :			
Level :		Lesson Duration :	

Lesson Objectives :

Sequence :

Props / Oils :

Music :

Quote:

" *My biggest struggles have been my biggest teachers* "

YOGA LESSON PLAN

Venue :		Date / Time :	
Lesson Plan Ref :			
Level :		Lesson Duration :	

Lesson Objectives :

Sequence :

Props / Oils :

Music :

Quote:

*" Calming the mind is yoga.
Not just standing on the head "*

YOGA LESSON PLAN

Venue :		Date / Time :	
Lesson Plan Ref :			
Level :		Lesson Duration :	

Lesson Objectives :

Sequence :

Props / Oils :

Music :

Quote:

"The body is your temple. Keep it pure and clean for the soul to reside in "

YOGA LESSON PLAN

Venue :		Date / Time :	
Lesson Plan Ref :			
Level :		Lesson Duration :	

Lesson Objectives :

Sequence :

Props / Oils :

Music :

Quote:

" Sometimes giving yourself a break
is th very thing you need "

YOGA LESSON PLAN

Venue :		Date / Time :	
Lesson Plan Ref :			
Level :		Lesson Duration :	

Lesson Objectives :

Sequence :

Props / Oils :	Music :

Quote:

" Yoga does not transform the way we see things, it transforms the person who sees "

YOGA LESSON PLAN

Venue :		Date / Time :	
Lesson Plan Ref :			
Level :		Lesson Duration :	

Lesson Objectives :

Sequence :

Props / Oils :	Music :

Quote:

" Yoga is the perfect opportunity to be curious about who you are "

YOGA LESSON PLAN

Venue :		Date / Time :	
Lesson Plan Ref :			
Level :		Lesson Duration :	

Lesson Objectives :

Sequence :

Props / Oils :	Music :

Quote:

" I bend so I don't break "

YOGA LESSON PLAN

Venue :		Date / Time :	
Lesson Plan Ref :			
Level :		Lesson Duration :	

Lesson Objectives :

Sequence :

Props / Oils :	Music :

Quote:

" Throw your hair in a bun, downward dog like a boss, and handle it "

YOGA LESSON PLAN

Venue :		Date / Time :	
Lesson Plan Ref :			
Level :		Lesson Duration :	

Lesson Objectives :

Sequence :

| Props / Oils : | Music : |

Quote:

" *Inhale the future, exhale the past* "

YOGA LESSON PLAN

Venue :		Date / Time :	
Lesson Plan Ref :			
Level :		Lesson Duration :	

Lesson Objectives :

Sequence :

Props / Oils :

Music :

Quote:

" The pose begins when you want to leave it "

YOGA LESSON PLAN

Venue :		Date / Time :	
Lesson Plan Ref :			
Level :		Lesson Duration :	

Lesson Objectives :

Sequence :

Props / Oils :	Music :

Quote:

" The longest journey of any person is the journey inward "

YOGA LESSON PLAN

Venue :		Date / Time :	
Lesson Plan Ref :			
Level :		Lesson Duration :	

Lesson Objectives :

Sequence :

Props / Oils :

Music :

Quote:

" Yoga is a mirror to look at ourselves from within "

YOGA LESSON PLAN

Venue :		Date / Time :	
Lesson Plan Ref :			
Level :		Lesson Duration :	

Lesson Objectives :

Sequence :

Props / Oils :	Music :

Quote:

" The yoga pose you avoid the most you need the most "

YOGA LESSON PLAN

Venue :		Date / Time :	
Lesson Plan Ref :			
Level :		Lesson Duration :	

Lesson Objectives :

Sequence :

Props / Oils :

Music :

Quote:

" Yoga is the journey of the self, through the self, to the self "

YOGA LESSON PLAN

Venue :		Date / Time :	
Lesson Plan Ref :			
Level :		Lesson Duration :	

Lesson Objectives :

Sequence :

Props / Oils :	Music :

Quote:

" Yoga is the fountain of youth. You've only as young as your spine is flexible "

YOGA LESSON PLAN

Venue :		Date / Time :	
Lesson Plan Ref :			
Level :		Lesson Duration :	

Lesson Objectives :

Sequence :

Props / Oils :	Music :

Quote:

" A flower does not think of competing to the flower next to it. It just blooms "

YOGA LESSON PLAN

Venue :		Date / Time :	
Lesson Plan Ref :			
Level :		Lesson Duration :	

Lesson Objectives :

Sequence :

Props / Oils :	Music :

Quote:

" Yoga exists in the world because everything is linked "

YOGA LESSON PLAN

Venue :		Date / Time :	
Lesson Plan Ref :			
Level :		Lesson Duration :	

Lesson Objectives :

Sequence :

Props / Oils :	Music :

Quote:

" Yoga. Because punching people is frowned upon."

YOGA LESSON PLAN

Venue :		Date / Time :	
Lesson Plan Ref :			
Level :		Lesson Duration :	

Lesson Objectives :

Sequence :

Props / Oils :	Music :

Quote:

" Yoga is not for the flexible. It's for th willing "

YOGA LESSON PLAN

Venue :		Date / Time :	
Lesson Plan Ref :			
Level :		Lesson Duration :	

Lesson Objectives :

Sequence :

Props / Oils :

Music :

Quote:

" For those wounded by civilization, yoga is the most healing salve "

YOGA LESSON PLAN

Venue :		Date / Time :	
Lesson Plan Ref :			
Level :		Lesson Duration :	

Lesson Objectives :

Sequence :

Props / Oils :	Music :

Quote:

" Yoga is the space where flower blossoms."

YOGA LESSON PLAN

Venue :		Date / Time :	
Lesson Plan Ref :			
Level :		Lesson Duration :	

Lesson Objectives :

Sequence :

Props / Oils :	Music :

Quote:

" Yoga is the cessation of the movements of the mind.
Then there is abiding in the Seer's own form."

YOGA LESSON PLAN

Venue :		Date / Time :	
Lesson Plan Ref :			
Level :		Lesson Duration :	

Lesson Objectives :

Sequence :

Props / Oils :	Music :

Quote:

" *The attitude of gratitude is the highest yoga.* "

YOGA LESSON PLAN

Venue :		Date / Time :	
Lesson Plan Ref :			
Level :		Lesson Duration :	

Lesson Objectives :

Sequence :

Props / Oils :

Music :

Quote:

" The soul is here for its own joy. "

YOGA LESSON PLAN

Venue :		Date / Time :	
Lesson Plan Ref :			
Level :		Lesson Duration :	

Lesson Objectives :

Sequence :

| Props / Oils : | Music : |
| | |

Quote:

" Yoga is 99% practice and 1% theory. "

YOGA LESSON PLAN

Venue :		Date / Time :	
Lesson Plan Ref :			
Level :		Lesson Duration :	

Lesson Objectives :

Sequence :

Props / Oils :	Music :

Quote:

" Here and now is where yoga begins "

YOGA LESSON PLAN

Venue :		Date / Time :	
Lesson Plan Ref :			
Level :		Lesson Duration :	

Lesson Objectives :

Sequence :

Props / Oils :	Music :

Quote:

" Yoga is not about self-improvement.
It's about self-acceptance."

YOGA LESSON PLAN

Venue :		Date / Time :	
Lesson Plan Ref :			
Level :		Lesson Duration :	

Lesson Objectives :

Sequence :

Props / Oils :	Music :

Quote:

" Yoga teaches us to cure what need not be endured and endure what cannot be cured "

YOGA LESSON PLAN

Venue :		Date / Time :	
Lesson Plan Ref :			
Level :		Lesson Duration :	

Lesson Objectives :

Sequence :

Props / Oils :

Music :

Quote:

" Sky above earth below peace within "

YOGA LESSON PLAN

Venue :		Date / Time :	
Lesson Plan Ref :			
Level :		Lesson Duration :	

Lesson Objectives :

Sequence :

Props / Oils :

Music :

Quote:

" The body benefits from movement, and the mind benefits from stillness "

YOGA LESSON PLAN

Venue :		Date / Time :	
Lesson Plan Ref :			
Level :		Lesson Duration :	

Lesson Objectives :

Sequence :

Props / Oils :	Music :

Quote:

" My biggest struggles have been my biggest teachers "

YOGA LESSON PLAN

Venue :		Date / Time :	
Lesson Plan Ref :			
Level :		Lesson Duration :	

Lesson Objectives :

Sequence :

Props / Oils :

Music :

Quote:

*" Calming the mind is yoga.
Not just standing on the head "*

YOGA LESSON PLAN

Venue :		Date / Time :	
Lesson Plan Ref :			
Level :		Lesson Duration :	

Lesson Objectives :

Sequence :

Props / Oils :	Music :

Quote:

"The body is your temple. Keep it pure and clean for the soul to reside in"

YOGA LESSON PLAN

Venue :		Date / Time :	
Lesson Plan Ref :			
Level :		Lesson Duration :	

Lesson Objectives :

Sequence :

Props / Oils :	Music :

Quote:

" Sometimes giving yourself a break is th very thing you need "

YOGA LESSON PLAN

Venue :		Date / Time :	
Lesson Plan Ref :			
Level :		Lesson Duration :	

Lesson Objectives :

Sequence :

Props / Oils :	Music :

Quote:

" Yoga does not transform the way we see things, it transforms the person who sees "

YOGA LESSON PLAN

Venue :		Date / Time :	
Lesson Plan Ref :			
Level :		Lesson Duration :	

Lesson Objectives :

Sequence :

Props / Oils :	Music :

Quote:

" Yoga is the perfect opportunity to be curious about who you are"

YOGA LESSON PLAN

Venue :		Date / Time :	
Lesson Plan Ref :			
Level :		Lesson Duration :	

Lesson Objectives :

Sequence :

Props / Oils :	Music :

Quote:

" I bend so I don't break "

YOGA LESSON PLAN

Venue :		Date / Time :	
Lesson Plan Ref :			
Level :		Lesson Duration :	

Lesson Objectives :

Sequence :

Props / Oils :

Music :

Quote:

" Throw your hair in a bun, downward dog like a boss, and handle it "

YOGA LESSON PLAN

Venue :		Date / Time :	
Lesson Plan Ref :			
Level :		Lesson Duration :	

Lesson Objectives :

Sequence :

Props / Oils :	Music :

Quote:

" Inhale the future, exhale the past "

YOGA LESSON PLAN

Venue :		Date / Time :	
Lesson Plan Ref :			
Level :		Lesson Duration :	

Lesson Objectives :

Sequence :

Props / Oils :	Music :

Quote:

" The pose begins when you want to leave it "

YOGA LESSON PLAN

Venue :		Date / Time :	
Lesson Plan Ref :			
Level :		Lesson Duration :	

Lesson Objectives :

Sequence :

Props / Oils :

Music :

Quote:

" The longest journey of any person is the journey inward "

YOGA LESSON PLAN

Venue :		Date / Time :	
Lesson Plan Ref :			
Level :		Lesson Duration :	

Lesson Objectives :

Sequence :

Props / Oils :

Music :

Quote:

" *Yoga is a mirror to look at ourselves from within* "

YOGA LESSON PLAN

Venue :		Date / Time :	
Lesson Plan Ref :			
Level :		Lesson Duration :	

Lesson Objectives :

Sequence :

Props / Oils :	Music :

Quote:

" The yoga pose you avoid the most you need the most "

YOGA LESSON PLAN

Venue :		Date / Time :	
Lesson Plan Ref :			
Level :		Lesson Duration :	

Lesson Objectives :

Sequence :

Props / Oils :

Music :

Quote:

" Yoga is the journey of the self, through the self, to the self "

YOGA LESSON PLAN

Venue :		Date / Time :	
Lesson Plan Ref :			
Level :		Lesson Duration :	

Lesson Objectives :

Sequence :

Props / Oils :	Music :

Quote:

" Yoga is the fountain of youth. You've only as young as your spine is flexible "

YOGA LESSON PLAN

Venue :		Date / Time :	
Lesson Plan Ref :			
Level :		Lesson Duration :	

Lesson Objectives :

Sequence :

Props / Oils :

Music :

Quote:

" A flower does not think of competing to the flower next to it. It just blooms "

YOGA LESSON PLAN

Venue :		Date / Time :	
Lesson Plan Ref :			
Level :		Lesson Duration :	

Lesson Objectives :

Sequence :

Props / Oils :	Music :

Quote:

" *Yoga exists in the world because everything is linked* "

YOGA LESSON PLAN

Venue :		Date / Time :	
Lesson Plan Ref :			
Level :		Lesson Duration :	

Lesson Objectives :

Sequence :

Props / Oils :

Music :

Quote:

" *Yoga. Because punching people is frowned upon.* "

YOGA LESSON PLAN

Venue :		Date / Time :	
Lesson Plan Ref :			
Level :		Lesson Duration :	

Lesson Objectives :

Sequence :

Props / Oils :	Music :

Quote:

" Yoga is not for the flexible. It's for th willing"

YOGA LESSON PLAN

Venue :		Date / Time :	
Lesson Plan Ref :			
Level :		Lesson Duration :	

Lesson Objectives :

Sequence :

Props / Oils :

Music :

Quote:

" For those wounded by civilization, yoga is the most healing salve "

YOGA LESSON PLAN

Venue :		Date / Time :	
Lesson Plan Ref :			
Level :		Lesson Duration :	

Lesson Objectives :

Sequence :

Props / Oils :	Music :

Quote:

" Yoga is the space where flower blossoms."

YOGA LESSON PLAN

Venue :		Date / Time :	
Lesson Plan Ref :			
Level :		Lesson Duration :	

Lesson Objectives :

Sequence :

Props / Oils :

Music :

Quote:

"Yoga is the cessation of the movements of the mind. Then there is abiding in the Seer's own form."

YOGA LESSON PLAN

Venue :		Date / Time :	
Lesson Plan Ref :			
Level :		Lesson Duration :	

Lesson Objectives :

Sequence :

Props / Oils :	Music :

Quote:

" The attitude of gratitude is the highest yoga. "

YOGA LESSON PLAN

Venue :		Date / Time :	
Lesson Plan Ref :			
Level :		Lesson Duration :	

Lesson Objectives :

Sequence :

Props / Oils :

Music :

Quote:

" The soul is here for its own joy. "

YOGA LESSON PLAN

Venue :		Date / Time :	
Lesson Plan Ref :			
Level :		Lesson Duration :	

Lesson Objectives :

Sequence :

Props / Oils :	Music :

Quote:

" Yoga is 99% practice and 1% theory. "

Made in United States
North Haven, CT
28 March 2023

34667712R00067